Natural Strength

Oscar Smith

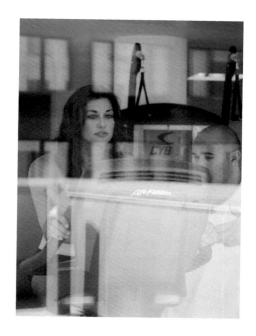

Oscar and Fit model Christina Trainer

TABLE OF CONTENTS

Dedication

To Nedra who always believed in me even

when I did not. Your words and knowledge

shaped me to be the man I am today.

You are always in my heart and soul.

FORWARD

Oscar Smith has inspired many of us over the years with his dedication to his clients and his authentic desire to see people evolve into better versions of themselves. Oscar is the owner of O-D studio (www.O-Dstudio.com) located in Tribeca, New York City.

His unique take on fitness and ability to create the right mindset is what allows his clients to actually have fun while they work out and has earned him an unmatched reputation as a certified personal trainer and gym owner. He is also a certified flexibility technician and has a strong background in kinesiology and biomechanics. His clientele has consisted of supermodels, celebrities and pro-athletes.

Not only has he coached his clients into excellent shape, but he has also dedicated his life to helping and rescuing people. He has served as a Grade 3 Ocean Lifeguard (16 years) and a NYPD Search and Rescue Diver (a position requiring so much physical fitness that only a handful of police officers has made the cut). Oscar is a former gymnast, and is currently a big wave bodysurfer, runner, and triathlete. He has been featured in Men's Health, W Magazine, GQ, and Shape Magazine, and has appeared on networks such as CNN, NBC, CBS, and Fox.

Oscar is really excited to publish this book so that he can get his message out to everyone. He understands that everyone has different fitness goals and wants to see people bring more passion and fun into their lives. He believes that finding physical activities and workouts that people can get excited about can give us more natural strength. I am proud to know Oscar and hope that his message can help you create a positive change in your life.

- Agnieszka (Oscar's wife)

THE CLIENT LIST

Let's get this out of the way. I know you are dying to know which celebrities and models I have trained over the past 14 years, so here is a list.

Celebrities:

Katherine Mcphee

Ed Burns

Tom Brady

Rosario Dawson

Val Kilmer

Amanda Bynes

David Blaine

Ryan Leslie

Tao Okamoto

Director Edgar Wright

Ryan Serhant (MDLNY on Bravo)

Jackie Cruz

Brain Vickers (Nascar #55)

Matt White (song writer/singer)

Ryan Cooper (actor/model)

James Blunt

Models:

Maryna Linchuk

Catherine McNeil

Anne Vyalitsyna

Hailey Clauson

Solange Wilvert

Kate Caune

Lina Sandberg

May Anderson

Anna J.

Heather Marks

Anais Mali

Lara Stone

Zuzanna Bijoch

Hannah Holman

Rianne Ten Haken

Louisa Taadou

Marlos Host

Julia Staigner

Petra Nemcova

Jessica Gomes

Selita Ebanks

Arizona Muse

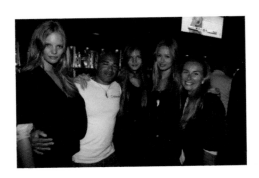

At a Justin Tuck event (linebacker for the NY Giants) with models Marlos Host, Mayara Rubik, Ania Cywińska, and Oscar's wife AgA

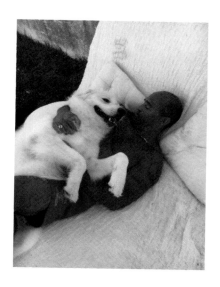

INTRODUCTION

Imagine yourself getting in really great shape, having more energy, more self-confidence and more fun. Too good to be true? Well it is not. When I was training to become a member on the U.S. Gymnastics Team, the words I never heard from my teammates were, "I can't." I learned an "I can do" mindset from some of the best athletes in the world and have carried this mental attitude with me in all aspects of my life.

I assume you are reading this book because you want to get in great shape and hear what an expert like me has to say about it, right? I will also assume you have picked up this book because other programs haven't worked. If they did work, you would probably be out there doing whatever it is that makes you look and feel great. Well, I want to let you know that you have come to the right place.

People come to me because they need help to achieve their personal fitness or health goals. There is no diet pill or quick workout that will give you lasting results. The results I offer my clients are real—but it requires hard work and sweat.

I'm really excited to share my secrets of success with you. As a personal trainer and fitness coach, I am very passionate about helping my clients get the results they desire. I'm proud to say that my clientele has consisted of all types of people in various professions, and I have helped all of them get into the best shape of their lives. My aim is to share with you the same things I share with my clients so that you can achieve your fitness goals —whatever they may be.

Natural strength is my own personal philosophy in regard to fitness and it's about strengthening your motivation, mind, and body. I believe that reaching your peak plateaus and overcoming them in fitness can only be attained if you find things that you naturally love to do. When you were a kid you were probably more active than you are now. Kids love to move around and play games; they also don't compartmentalize exercise in their minds.

I'm here to tell you that if you reconnect with that inner child, you will be able to maximize your workouts and have more fun in the process of getting healthy. I believe that a balanced approach to fitness that honors our inner child can help us find more happiness and feel more fulfilled.

I notice a lot of people becoming fanatics when they start to get in shape. I don't believe you need to become a gym rat or yoga junkie. It's just not necessary. Working out doesn't have to take over your whole life, but if it helps you to stay a little bit more healthy and less stressed, that's awesome!

What I want you to realize before you begin to try some of my tips and workouts is that there is no magic fad diet or workout regimen that is going to get you into shape in 2 –3 weeks. It just doesn't work that way. In my experience as a trainer, I see that the human body loses fat in certain areas first and that it takes people about 2 –3 months of healthier eating and working out to get the results they want.

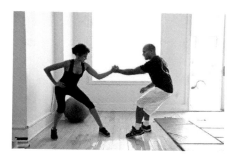

Oscar and Ford model Cici Ali

Don't be discouraged by this —it's really not that long of a wait to give yourself what you really desire. In addition, if you work on changing your mindset you will create a lifestyle change that is different than a specific exercise or diet fad. The following section, *Mindset*, is going to talk about this more.

My program can help you increase strength because I am going to encourage you to increase your endurance, balance, and coordination. Unlike other trainers, my training methods aim to tone the entire body, giving you more power and the ability to perform in sports and real life activities.

Working on increasing your overall strength doesn't just make you look and feel better, it also has health benefits. It reduces sarcopenia (the loss of muscle mass due to aging) and slows down the aging process in general. Developing a lifestyle of working out will help you stay agile as you age and allow you to retain your power and muscle mass so that you can continue to do activities you enjoy.

In this book I have put together all of my greatest tips and workouts from my 25 years of experience as an athlete and a personal trainer. My hope for you is that you can look at these workouts and pick out a few to try for yourself. Check out my program in the last section of this book (*6 Weeks to a Beach Body)* if you really want to get serious.

I have designed several different types of workouts for you to try. You can join a gym (which these days are priced pretty reasonably), but you don't have to. Many people can get the same results by working out at home and getting outdoors. You can easily create a home gym by investing in some equipment like a pull-up bar, exercise ball, jump rope, dumbbells, and more. A lot of people don't have access to a nearby gym or don't want to pay the monthly fees. That is why I have designed and categorized these workouts for you to take to places like the park, the beach, and the pool. I have also designed workouts for your home, hotel room, and office. Basically, I want you to create a mindset in which you look forward to working out wherever you are.

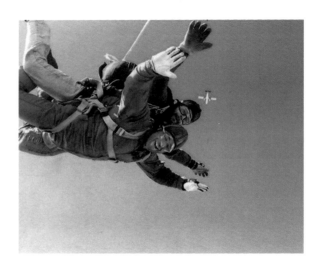

HOW I GOT STARTED

I love working out and have always been an athlete. As a kid, I was always active and involved in sports like football and track and field. I couldn't imagine a life without exercise because it makes me happy. It's my lifestyle and I sustain it by making it fun. However, keeping myself fit has not just been for vanity's sake, but has helped me save people's lives through the jobs and careers I have chosen.

Not only have I been an ocean lifeguard, but I've also spent time as a NYPD Search and Rescue Diver in the Special Operations Division (SOD). We are basically SWAT on water, and our training is intense. I graduated from the police academy and did five years of regular patrol time (car stops, made arrests, and of course gave out traffic tickets). I was also a detective.

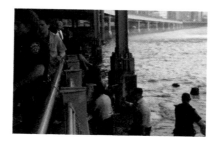

Oscar doing an arrest underneath the Brooklyn Bridge

After you are seasoned, you can put in for other things like scuba. You have to be picked according to your expertise—mine was water.

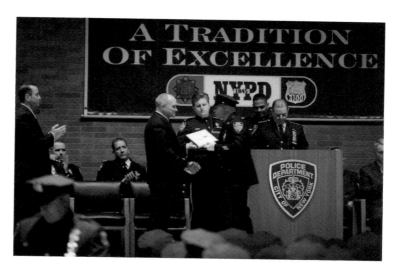

Promotion to Detective

Out of 40,000 New York City cops, I am proud to say I was one of 30 on the Search and Rescue Team. Lots of people and things end up in the miles of waterways in New York, and the Rescue Team assists in these situations. Imagine jumping out of a helicopter strapped with over 150lbs of gear in order to drag a terrified person out of the water in winter, searching for bombs during the United Nations General Assembly, or protecting the President when he lands at the Wall Street Heliport—the list goes on. It was tough but also extremely rewarding.

When US Airways Flight 1549 had to make an emergency landing in the Hudson River, we were there to help. The ferries had come to rescue all the passengers within minutes, but it was our team, the Special Operations Division, that came in to secure the plane so that it wouldn't sink or float down the river and end up near the Statue of Liberty jetting out of the shallow water (which would have been quite a sight).

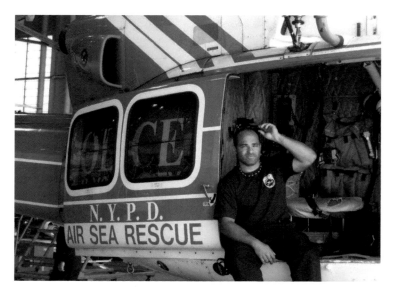

The scuba team also had to double check that no bodies were inside. Luckily, no one lost their lives. The water was freezing (32–35 degrees Fahrenheit) and we had to babysit the plane for 2–3 days until a crane could come and haul it away. When I came home the next day my wife literally said my lips were purple.

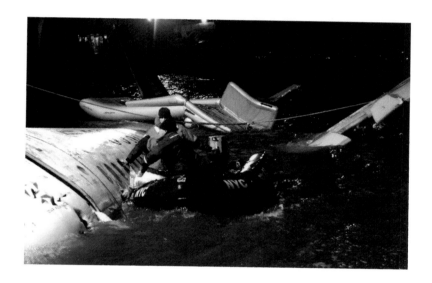

I realized when I was young that my body would be my profession. I was inspired to become a personal trainer in 1991 when I was working at a law office and attending college. I was also a gymnast at the time and my dream was to make it on the US Olympic Gymnastics Team. I was pretty busy. The '92 Summer Olympics were coming up and I was in great shape.

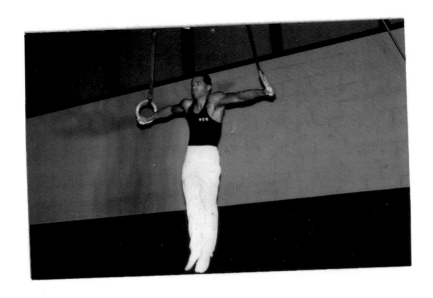

I was working the night shift at the gym when a guy came up to me and said, "Hey, can I work out with you?" I thought this was a really strange request. I didn't know him and nobody had asked me that before. He said, "I want to train with you because I want to look the way you do—so I want to do what you do." He then explained to me what a personal trainer was.

Back then, personal trainers were more obscure. You only heard about them because people like Tom Cruise, Madonna, and Oprah had one. I gave him a weird look because it seemed like a high prestigious thing to me. He said, "Look, I'll pay you just to come follow you around when you work out." That got my attention. I thought, "This is interesting." And this was how I got the idea of becoming a personal trainer.

I started talking to the physical therapists and trainers at my college to see what their backgrounds were. I ended up meeting some amazing guys in the field. One guy was Frank Hunter (Nassau Community College) who became a close mentor of mine and who was a former trainer for the US Olympic team. I also met some of the key Jet players in the 90's like Mark Gastineau and Joe Klecko. The Jets training camp was just down the road from the college. Nassau was known as The Football Factory back then.

The pros inspired me and kept me focused on my goals. The bodybuilder/powerlifters and other big-time pros would poke some fun at me, but Frank would say to them, "Pound per pound, Oscar is stronger than you guys ever will be." This was because my body mass index (BMI) just wasn't as high. He would have me demonstrate how I could lay on the floor with my arms stretched out in front and push up to a standing position. I was incredibly strong but also lean, which helped me when it came to doing gymnastics and other sports.

In life there are moments when everything changes for you. For me that moment was in Long Beach, New York, when I was 23 years old. I was doing personal training on the side, while also working at a law office because I thought I would eventually become a lawyer.

I bumped into an old friend on the boardwalk. It was a hot summer day and he was in shorts with a lifeguard t-shirt on. I was feeling sweaty and constricted in a suit and tie. He told me about how much fun he was having as a beach lifeguard. I said, "Oh man, my job sucks. I'm waking up early and pulling boring cases all day and getting coffee for the office."

I loved to swim and thought about what it would be like to be on the beach every day—it sounded awesome. It wasn't soon after that that I thought, "What the hell?" I applied in the spring of 1989 to the city of Long Beach to be a lifeguard and was accepted. It was, however, competitive to join and get certain spots on the patrol. Below are some pictures of the competitions.

The chief of lifeguards realized what an asset I would be to them. I wasn't the fastest swimmer but I was a big strong guy and could help out in rescues. Lifeguarding was great because it was like being a professional athlete.

From 9–11 a.m. every day we worked out. We had to run, swim, and do practice rescues. By the end of the summer, I was in fantastic shape. I realize now that my body type helped me to be more approachable as a trainer. I wasn't a bodybuilder but I was super fit and people saw my methods as more attainable for them.

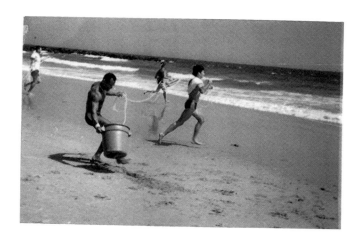

After 13 years of being a personal trainer part-time, I ended up opening my own training studio in 2003—O-D Studio in Manhattan. My personal training program consists of interval training (cardio and strength training), weight training, boxing/kickboxing, yoga, Pilates, and flexibility training. I aim to help people target every area of the body and look the best they possibly can. If you do decide to work with a personal trainer, it's really important that they keep your workouts diverse. This has been one of the keys to my success as a trainer.

Early on, O-D Studio started to attract models because some of the Victoria's Secret models, who lived directly across the street, wandered into my gym. I got them into great shape while providing them with a comfortable and authentic energy that they told me was a breath of fresh air (coming from the fashion industry). Plus, my studio was a private studio where they wouldn't be recognized or bothered by anyone. Word quickly caught on amongst other models that my gym was a terrific place to get into optimal shape. The competitive nature of the girls brought a ton of business into the studio. Celebrities in the neighborhood soon followed suit and started coming in.

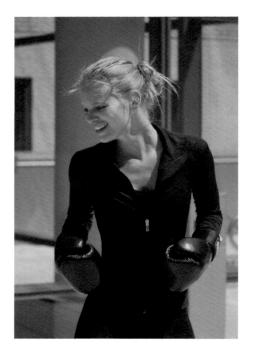

Model Marlos Host

Celebrity clients don't just find me in a Google search. My work with celebrities, models, and pro-athletes has spread through word of mouth and I take my business very seriously. I am proud of the results I deliver to clients.

I always ask my clients to tell me what kind of experiences they have had with athletics or personal training in the past. Those who have played sports as kids usually know what it is like to be coached. The truth is we don't get better in the arena of fitness without some coaching from someone who knows what they are doing. So I want you to think of this book as your own personal coach.

However, I'm not a coach that is going to yell at you and make you feel bad about yourself. This is because I know that this method doesn't work very well. Having a supportive trainer works much better. The people that are successful with exercise have found passions and activities that they love. If you have failed at a fitness plan in the past, consider that it didn't inspire you. We do enough work as it is. Who decided that working out ought to be a second job? Natural strength is about finding your passions so that you can create a more active lifestyle change. I want this book to be a hopeful message in your life.

I'm going to break down for you what works well when it comes to getting in shape. The three concepts I want you to hang onto as you read this book are:

Motivation. Your motivation is the reason you are reading this book. Motivation has to do with your passions and your goals. What's going to motivate you to really sweat?

Diversity. Diversity is a concept that separates me from other personal trainers. I want you to switch up your routines and try different things all the time. This will also keep your mind more engaged because you'll be having more fun.

Commitment. Your commitment is about your dedication to a lifestyle change.

In this book I'm going to help you with the following:

* Reflect on your goals (which will be different for everybody).

* Assess your current mindset and envision your new lifestyle.

And Finally:

* The meat of this book—my own personal workouts for you to try.

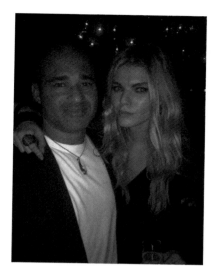

Oscar and model Maryna Linchuk at Victoria's Secret show after party

MINDSET

There are a lot of fad diets and fitness programs out there and many people fail with these programs. The Exercise Industrial Complex (my term for all the trainers, gyms, and companies with products on infomercials) is a multi-billion-dollar industry. Truth be told, they don't care if you fail or succeed—they just love putting the newest program out and getting you to buy it.

Around the New Year, people sign up for gym memberships, seeking to turn over a new leaf, but often give up around February. People who fail at these programs are often missing an important piece to the puzzle: play.

In my training, I have a philosophy that emphasizes finding the inner child within each of us. It's my belief that we can get pretty disconnected from ourselves, our bodies, and each other in our culture. I believe that in order to find our natural strength, we need to find our inner child. It might sound cheesy, but hear me out—this philosophy has helped me maintain my athleticism and motivate countless clients in their workout practices.

Our Inner Child Vs. Our Adult Mind

When I train with clients, I do workouts with them ranging from 1–3 hours. I know that may seem long, but remember, I am getting pro-athletes, models, and celebrities into prime shape. I came up with the idea of getting in touch with the inner child when I asked people how long they usually worked out for.

They would say, "I don't know, 45 minutes to an hour max." I started to question where they got that idea.

Clients would tell me, "I don't know, it's just the average that most people work out."

I said, "When you were a kid you would go outside and play 4, 6, 8 hours at a time. You would play full games of basketball, baseball, or whatever your sport was. As a kid, you didn't see it as exercise—you thought of it as having fun."

Why is that? When kids play, they are enjoying the moment, releasing energy, laughing and challenging themselves. I started to understand that adults compartmentalize physical activity as a certain thing, like going to the gym for 45 minutes every other day. Children, on the other hand, do activities and sports with their friends and see it as playing. And because they are having a fun, social interaction, they are actually able to get better, longer workouts. Don't get me wrong, I think it's great if you can get to the gym 45 minutes every other day. However, when I look at people who are exercising for hours at a time—people doing triathlons or running marathons—there are two things to realize about their success:

1. They are at a fun event.

2. They are surrounded by people aspiring to be great athletes.

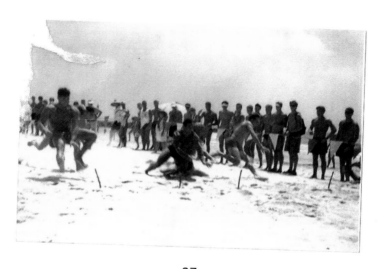

Being around others is a key component to getting into this kind of a zone. I'm not saying you should make it your goal to start with such long activities. I actually want you to start with easier goals and work your way up to more, especially if you haven't exercised in a while. What I am saying is that we need to understand that motivation and having fun plays a huge role in our level of endurance.

Now let's fast forward. If we, as adults, try to get our friends together to do a day-long game of basketball or baseball, it's pretty much impossible. Everyone is too busy. However, I would argue that deep down everyone wants to embrace the kid inside—to play, jump, run around, and be silly.

The truth is that people aren't even that connected anymore. You go to the beach and look around and lots of people are on their smartphones instead of taking in the beautiful day. Becoming conscious of our mindset and where we are at is really important. If you are feeling disconnected from life in general, I want to encourage you to think about the energy you had when you were a kid so that you can learn to bring that energy into your adult life and cultivate your natural strength.

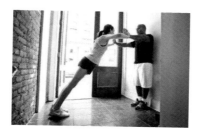

Oscar with Ford model JP

MOTIVATION

I'm a great person to take advice from because of two things:

1. I have had a ton of success as an athlete and as a personal trainer.

2. I understand that not everybody who wants to be healthier or in better shape is or ever has been an athlete.

I get that your motivation may be different than mine or one of my pro-athlete clients and that's perfectly fine. In addition, I realize that not everyone played on sports teams or was ever physically active when they were younger. Either way, I want you to use your motivation to come up with some realistic goals for yourself.

Try New Things

Finding your natural strength is dependent on feeling motivated and inspired. If you want some of that energy and joy you felt when you were a kid, you have to find things that you love to do. Step out of your comfort zone and try something new.

Create goals based on what you want to achieve and what will make you happy. I would argue that happiness is really about finding joy in simple things. If it's a nice day, try getting outside and going for a bike ride, a hike in the forest, some Tai Chi in the park, or a walk. Dogs are great because they motivate us to be more active. Getting fresh air is also really important. A lot of senior citizens benefit from taking their dogs outside.

Does climbing a tree make you happy? Great! Washing your car on a Saturday afternoon? I'll count that as physical activity as it gets you outside and moving. It also releases endorphins and adrenaline. If you are a busy working professional, try killing two birds with one stone by walking to the grocery store and carrying your groceries back—a form of weight training. Also, little things like taking the stairs instead of the elevator, or riding your bike instead of driving, add up over time.

Hobbies keep us active too. Hobbies like woodworking or home construction projects are actually pretty physically demanding. People who do these things have a lot of natural strength, especially in the upper body. They are used to lifting all kinds of materials. I remember when I was in high school; a classmate's father did construction. He was able to pick up 4x4s with his hands, which were like vice grips. This came from lifting bags of cement and buckets full of materials all day.

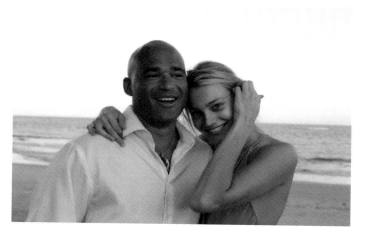

Oscar with model Anna J.

Social Interaction

Another aspect to staying motivated is having social interaction with other people. Let's say you are a gardener (which is a great low impact activity). You get to be active, build up your muscles, break a sweat, and receive the joy of watching something grow. In addition, you may get praise and compliments from your neighbors as they notice how great your garden looks. This, in turn, would give you a warm feeling inside, which would make you more inspired to keep at it.

Studies have shown that people are addicted to social media. Why? Because we get a lot of acknowledgement from other people. You post a picture and you get a ton of likes. It feels good. However, social media is a poor substitute for face-to-face human interaction. Additionally, social media actually seems to make people more isolated and depressed overall because it's not based in reality. This is why I think that any activity you do that helps you spark up a conversation with another person is important.

One thing missing from many people's lives is play. A lot of people don't have the social skills to reach out and talk to people. You don't even see many kids at the park playing games like tag anymore. These days, we play more games on our phones. But exercising our socialization muscle is important because other people can help keep us motivated to work out.

If you are a member of a fitness gym, I challenge you to learn the names of the people at the front desk. Think about walking into a gym where people know your name. It has a different vibe to it than walking into a room full of strangers. And subconsciously you will start to feel that the gym is a more welcoming environment and that it feels good to be there. This is really based on the principle that you get what you give. Exercising your socialization muscle may even lead to things like playing games in the park with other people or finding a tennis partner to play matches with. This is also the reason why I created an app called FITBUD (www.thefitbudapp.com).

Goals

Here are some examples of goals my clients tell me they want to attain:

* Have more energy

* Not be winded when I play with my kids

* Reduce my medications

* Have more fun

* Find activities I love to do

* Feel stronger and more toned

* Lose weight

* Eat better

* Reduce stress and improve focus

* Lower high blood pressure

* Be more confident

* Look and feel better

Find something you enjoy doing; start slowly and increase your weekly goals as you build up your strength and endurance. You don't want to hurt yourself. Issues like tendonitis and various back injuries are common.

I explain to people that when I go out and bodysurf hurricane waves, it is not something I just decided to do; it took me years to build up the strength to surf those waves. I see the following happening all the time: someone who wants to get in better shape sees someone really fit doing something either on TV, at the gym, or in a yoga class. They say to themselves, "If I want to look like that person I'd better do that too," and inevitably end up hurting themselves because they have not built up to it. People often feel like they don't ever want to work out again after they hurt themselves. I don't want this to be your experience, and I also don't want your goals to be so large that you burn out after a week or so.

Starting Out

I can already hear you asking me, "Oscar, what should I do and how much should I do it?" This all depends on your past experience with working out. Do you like fishing? Yoga? Standing on your head? Go for it! Any activity that makes you feel good is a great place to start. If you join a gym, try basic things like walking on a treadmill, riding the stationary bike, or participating in a couple of classes. I always recommend trying the weight machines, but keeping it simple when you are beginning.

Gyms are great places to work out, but I don't believe gyms are for everyone—in fact, I know some people who find them boring and monotonous. If you are one of these people, my advice to you is to find something else to do. Maybe yoga, tennis, swimming laps, or joining a running club will inspire you more. I just want to see you be healthy. I always ask my clients, "If you could add 10 years to your life, would you?" Well, this is exactly what exercise has been scientifically proven to do. It keeps you healthy so that you can live your life to the fullest.

The human body is a machine similar to a car. We all know that if you leave a car in a garage for months or years without driving it, the car will start to decay. The valves and belts will corrode from lack of movement and lubrication. It's the same concept with the human body: if you don't get it going, you may start to see health issues.

Sometimes I hear people say they feel too old to begin exercising, but I want to tell you something: you aren't too old, and adding some exercise into your life can really help with the aging process. I recommend starting with low impact activities like walking, swimming, or biking. I know that a lot of people at the age of 40 are already on several prescription medications for high blood pressure, cholesterol, diabetes etc. I would argue that if you just did a simple workout for 45 minutes to an hour every other day, it would greatly improve your health, and you may find that your doctor might tell you that you don't need certain medications anymore, or that you can cut some back.

Exercise:

What are your goals? How can you incorporate the concept of play into them? Write them down on a piece of paper and hang it up somewhere. No goal is too big or small. Your goals will help you stay motivated as you begin to examine your mindset. Don't hurt or overwhelm yourself. Start with small goals and increase them as you begin to cultivate more natural strength.

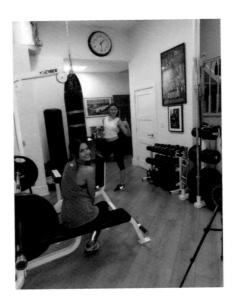

Models Adrianna Bach and Olga Kaboulova at Oscar's gym

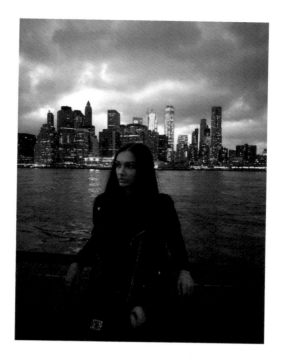

Model Weronika Banka

ROADBLOCKS

As a personal trainer I condition the human body. However, I also understand that conditioning the mind is imperative. If we don't have the proper mindset when trying to adapt a lifestyle change, we will fail. Why? Because we give up, often right before we would have started to see results. I don't want this to happen to you. That is why I want you to take some time to reflect on any mental roadblocks you may have to getting in shape. Maybe you tried a fitness program in the past and it didn't work for you, so now you don't believe it is possible for you to get in shape.

Adapting this program of natural strength means you are going to have to push yourself. It also means you are going to have to look at areas of your life that are not working. Being organized is a crucial aspect of making a new workout regimen stick around, and not be another fad. I want you to become conscious of your time management, cleanliness, and your ability to plan ahead. Maybe preparing meals ahead of time is the only thing that will prevent you from eating slices of pizza on your lunch break. In order to give yourself what you need, you need to be able to get organized—mentally, as well as physically.

Common Roadblocks

Time. Many people say they have no time. However, if you don't take care of yourself your health will demand your time. When my clients tell me they have limited time to work out, I always ask, "What time do you get up in the morning?" Getting healthy means you may have to get up an hour earlier so that you can do one of my half-hour workouts before you start your day. This may also mean that you need to get into bed an hour earlier.

I recommend this because many people say they are too exhausted to work out at the end of the day. Think about ways in which you can maximize your time and reorganize your schedule in order to fit your workouts in.

Another issue people have is that they are too busy with their kids or families. I believe bringing a childlike play into your fitness life is part of a healthy mindset. Therefore, find outdoor activities or games you can do with your family, friends, and your dogs. Go for a walk or ride bikes with them. It's important to honor these activities as valuable and understand that these simple things actually can help change your life. And guess what? Your family, friends, and dogs need the exercise too.

Feeling Overwhelmed. I hear a lot of people say they feel, "too out of shape to even start." A lot of people see images of super fit people exercising and then begin to feel overwhelmed even before beginning. Why is that? Your mind perceives a mountain of work and effort between what you desire and your perception of where you are. And sure, if working out for you is going to be a monotonous thing that is extremely difficult and joyless, it could feel like a mountain. However, I want you to move away from this kind of thinking because another reality is that you can enjoy your exercise and actually create a new way of approaching fitness that can benefit all areas of your life and make you feel more fulfilled all around. Doesn't that sound better and more achievable? Sure this will be a journey, but think of it more as a positive one rather than a treacherous one in which you really don't believe you will attain your goals.

Feeling Discouraged. If we focus primarily on the way we look rather than the way we feel, we may become discouraged before we even begin. If I could communicate only one thing to you, it would be that cultivating natural strength is a process that takes time. Paradoxically, we only have today. You must make it your goal to incorporate some fitness into each day, and begin the practice of noticing how you feel after you work out. Clients I work with tell me they love the feeling after a good workout—the feeling of being sore and physically exerted. This physical exertion releases adrenaline, endorphins, and relieves stress.

It also has a wide range of health benefits that I will discuss in the following section. Make these other aspects of natural strength important and it will help you to stay encouraged.

BIG Goals. We get overwhelmed when we set huge, lofty goals. I want you to focus on cultivating natural strength and feeling healthy overall. Eat better because it makes you feel better. Enjoy seeing weight drop off as a by-product rather than making that your number one goal.

Creating a lasting change means you need to be excited about it. When we do workouts we find boring, we burn out and are unable to make it a lifestyle. However, when you find things you like to do in supportive environments, these mental roadblocks will naturally taper down. Believe it or not, but you will get to the point where you look forward to working out. You will enjoy seeing your strength improve, and your mood will elevate.

Staying Positive. Pay attention to that critical inner voice. As a trainer, I see a lot of people weighed down by their own critical internal dialogue. Know that positive self-talk is a lot more effective in cultivating natural mental and physical strength than negative self-talk. Notice if you beat yourself up for missing a day or not achieving your goals as fast as you would like. That kind of mentality is something a lot of people get stuck in and it comes from a perfectionist, results-driven culture. It is also what makes people give up too soon. What our minds and bodies really need is a break from that mentality and to step into a realm that is fun, encouraging, and not so much about perfection.

Tips for Overcoming Roadblocks:

1. Get out of your comfort zone.

2. Get more social. Find a gym buddy. Join a club so that you can enjoy something physical with other people. Other people will help you get up and get out of the house.

3. Put down your phone. Don't be afraid to say hello to someone and learn people's names. Going to a gym with friendly people will get you to come back.

4. Utilize your resources. The internet is a great resource for information. You can look up workout routines, or find

activities going on in your community. Take this book with you when you go to the pool, the beach or the park. I wrote this book so that working out could be more accessible to you wherever you are. (This is also the reason why I created The FITBUD app and OD32 app).

Exercise:

What are your roadblocks? They'll be different for everyone. I encourage you to take a mental inventory and write them down. Hang them up if you want. *Post It* notes are great and use the magnet on the fridge. This will help you to stay more conscious of your mindset and be honest with yourself about where you are at mentally

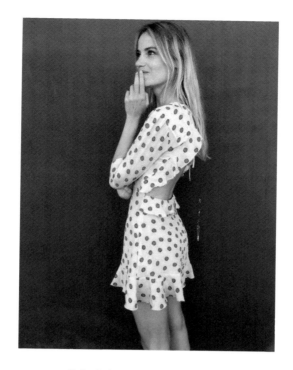

Model Tessa Westerhof

DIVERSITY

I always say do something different every day. It confuses the body. It's really easy to get bored with a monotonous routine. From my 25 years of experience, I know how important it is to try to mix it up and do different variations. I use a lot of different things, including my background with gymnastics, surfing, and Muay Thai.

I had great success as an athlete and trainer because I know how to make working out fun by maintaining a strong aspect of play and diversity. This is also what makes me different from a lot of other personal trainers out there. I encourage you to train in circuits and be very focused (don't be checking your email every five minutes). Learn how to *stay* focused and keep your heart rate up so that you can burn more calories and achieve your goals.

Doing your sets in waves—one set light, one heavy, one light, one heavy—will help you build strength and avoid a plateau. If you run a mile every day, eventually that mile will feel like a walk around the block. If however, you mix it up (try jumping rope, biking, or swimming) your body will get stronger.

I look up to Bruce Lee as an example of this. He studied Kung Fu, but he also developed his own style called Jeet Kune Do. Bruce developed this style after feeling like the traditional Chinese martial art form Wing Chun made a fight last too long and that it wasn't practical for a real street fight. He started to think outside the box and developed Jeet Kune Do, which utilizes many different training methods including running, endurance, flexibility, and incorporated activities such as fencing and boxing.

Bruce Lee has been my inspiration to develop my own style of training which incorporates:

* Weight training

* Mat work (Pilates)

* Strength training

* Core work

* Cardio training

* Interval training

* Agility

* Yoga and flexibility

* Stand-up boxing

* Kickboxing

* Plyometics

* HIT training (high intensity training)

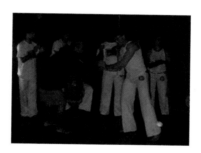

Oscar getting schooled in Brazilian Capoeira in Rio, Brazil

I do a lot of strength training and core work. I find it works best to mix up daily what I take clients through. A client will come in one day and we will do standup boxing. The next day abs. The next day plyometrics or some mat work (Pilates). I also incorporate weight training for both men and women.

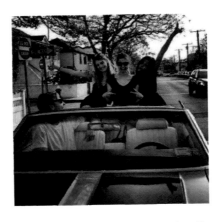

Models Tessa, Ophélie and Aline

COMMITMENT

Once you get out of the house, commit to going for it. If you are a swimmer, you know that once you get into the water you'll be cold. What's the fastest way to warm up? Swim! You are already wet, so you might as well. I think it's the same thing for just getting out of your house to do something active. If you open that front door, commit to doing something healthy for yourself (even if it's just a walk around the block for some fresh air).

Commitment is imperative to success and is about your dedication to this process. Your commitment to a lifestyle change is your commitment to yourself. You have to commit to working on respecting yourself, doing self-care, and getting healthy. No one is perfect at this, which is why I say commit to working on it.

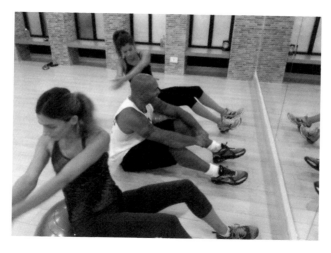

Oscar with owners of TrainStation Gym Rafa and Hiba in Beirut, Lebanon

HEALTH BENEFITS

When you exercise, your body releases adrenaline and endorphins, which helps to elevate your mood. It also increases your energy. The strongest drug in the world is adrenaline. We cannot fabricate it; we have tried. Even synthetic adrenaline is not the same as the one secreted from the adrenal gland in our brain. That's where we get that happy feeling or burst of energy after we start exercising. It's also where people get their superhuman strength in crisis situations. Working out is the only thing that can give you a steady dose of these powerful natural drugs that benefit your health.

The following is a list of health benefits reaped from exercising. I always recommend you see a doctor and get some bloodwork done. That is something I do regularly.

Seeing where your cholesterol numbers are at, for example, can help you make different decisions about your diet. I especially recommend seeing a doctor when you begin exercising if you have any health issues. Getting bloodwork done regularly can be another great way to measure your progress.

Benefits:

* Improved strength

* Better sleep

* Increase your daily metabolism

* Prevent back injuries

* Increase flexibility

* Weight loss

* Increase endurance and stamina

* Strengthen bones and joints

* Helps with aging process

* Reduce stress and strengthen resilience

* Balances hormones and lifts mood

* Decreases your risk of injury

* Regulate blood pressure and cholesterol

* Regulate diabetes

Exercise Reduces the Following Risks:

* Heart Disease**

* Diabetes

* Osteoporosis

* High blood pressure

* Obesity

** The heart is a muscle, so increasing your exercise regimen strengthens your heart's ability to pump more blood through the body. A person who exercises has a slower resting heart rate than someone that doesn't because their heart is performing better.

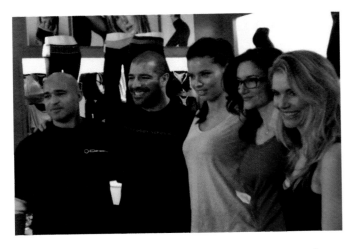

Oscar with model Adriana Lima and fitness trainers
Will Torres, Terri Walsh, and Kristin McGee

NUTRITION

Find out what works well with your body. Food is very individual and I don't recommend any specific way to eat. I do recommend removing a lot of junk food and processed food from your diet. Processed food is filled with chemicals and toxins that are difficult for your body to break down. I also tell people to limit the amount they drink and smoke because that will negatively affect your fitness process. I always say its 50 percent exercise and 50 percent food. If you don't see results in two to three months, you're doing something wrong.

You don't have to have a paleo or vegetarian diet, but make sure you're getting a lot of veggies, fruits, nuts, and nothing too rich. Be willing to make changes in your diet if you aren't seeing the results you want in about four weeks. Talk to a nutritionist if you need more assistance. Check out my last section in this book called, *What to Eat.*

Nutrition Tips:

* Snack on some protein (like a shake) before you lift.

* Eat about 30 minutes after you work out and not before (you don't want to be mopping up your meal).

* Don't eat too much— try smaller portions. Cut your calories in half and you will burn more than you take in.

* Protein is great after a workout. I recommend whey protein for making shakes, etc. However, keep in mind that protein is turned into and stored as fat when you cannot use it so do not overdo it.

* I recommend lots of lean chicken, fish, eggs, milk, whole grains, veggies, fruits, and nuts.

* Limit your carb intake if you are trying to lose weight (bread and refined sugar).

* No eating past 8 p.m.

* Drink plenty of water and/or juice to flush your system.

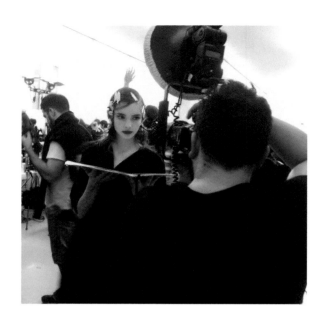

Model Paulina Frankowska

WORKOUT TIPS

Preventing Injury

You may have good intentions when you start working out with a super challenging program, but if you aren't conditioned for it you could wind up hurting yourself. It may be beneficial to work out with a personal trainer to help you practice proper form. Start off slow and pace yourself.

Workout Journal

People often fail at their workout plans because they are disorganized. It's easy to lose momentum when you are not keeping track of what you are doing. I recommend you keep a workout journal to track what you do each day, especially if you are doing weight or strength training. Start with committing to tracking at least eight weeks. It takes this much time to really start to see results. You also need to keep track of the amount of weight you are using and the number of sets and reps you are doing.

Warming Up

Always warm up with some cardio before you do resistance or strength training. Just warming up for 3–5 minutes with some light cardio is sufficient. I recommend doing some stretches after you warm up.

Cardio

Cardio is the fastest way to lose weight but you have to keep making it harder for maximum results. You will also get in better shape faster if you vary your cardio workouts. If you have had any joint issues, you can try low impact activities like biking or swimming. If you have issues with asthma, try taking it slow and walking up a hill or some stairs (biking is also good). The benefit of working out in the morning is that you will have more energy throughout the day.

Strength and Resistance Training

Strength and resistance training (also weight training) is a great way to stay toned, and to maintain or improve muscle and bone strength. It is also important for staying healthy as we age. You can use progressively heavier weights or challenges to improve strength. Make sure you have proper form before beginning to do sets of resistance training. Don't force yourself by doing too much too soon. Every day incorporate a little cardio so you don't hurt yourself, and give your body time to rest and recover

Practice good form by starting with low or no weight and doing slow movements. It's always a good idea to work with a trainer, coach, or someone who knows what they are doing so they can give you feedback.

Watch out for the following, as it will indicate incorrect form:

1. Anything that hurts once you start.

2. If it feels like you are working the wrong muscles.

3. Jerky or forced reps where you lose your form or center of balance.

Organizing strength and resistance training into 1–5 sets and doing 3–15 reps per set is standard (you can check out my strength training formulas in the following section, *The*

Exercises). A good rule of thumb is that the last two reps of a set should be pretty challenging. If it's not, you need to increase the weight or do more reps. If it's too challenging, you need to decrease the weight or do fewer reps.

Changing up the tempo of the speed at which you lift is a positive thing that can help work your muscles out in different ways. A lot of people do their reps fast, but try slowing them down once in a while. Pay attention to how much you rest between sets. If you do a lot of reps, the weight is less and your resting period can be shorter. If you do fewer reps the weight is probably higher and you will need to rest more in between sets. The time you need to rest is also a good way to measure your progress and something you can track in a journal.

Agonist and antagonist (positive/negative) muscle groups work together to push and pull our muscles. Make sure you are working both of these groups out so that one doesn't become stronger than the other (putting you out of balance). An example is when doing bench presses. Using the row machine would be beneficial as it would work the opposite muscle group (push/pull). And of course, if you use proper form, your core muscles should be engaged, giving you a better workout.

Don't be afraid to switch it up and do something completely different like yoga or HIT training after a lot of resistance training. Give yourself at least 24 hours of rest before repeating so your muscle groups can heal. Work out different muscles in the meantime (abs or core).

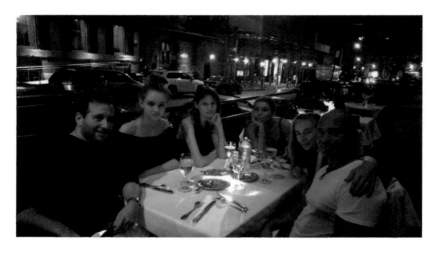

Dinner at Mr. Chow after the tommy show NYFW 2016

Tips for safety:

* Make sure you are rested before you work out.

* Stay hydrated.

* Warm up with some cardio for 3–5 minutes before you get into anything intense.

* Stretch after your warm-up. You don't want to stretch cold muscles. Also stretch after you finish your workout.

* Stop if you are getting any signals from your body such as: pain, extreme fatigue, etc.

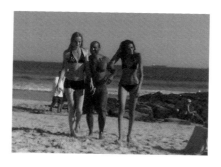

Oscar with the Ford models Simonee
from Brazil and Paula from Poland

THE EXERCISES

I'm excited to share with you these exercise programs
which have taken me years to perfect. I want you to realize
that I haven't just trained supermodels and athletes, but all
types of people. I make up custom routines for everyone—be
sure to check out the next section, *O-D STUDIO'S Featured
Workouts*. In this section, I have created various workouts for
specific clients ranging from a rabbi to a busy mom. In
addition, I have tried every one of my routines so I know how
hard or easy they are.

I know you might not know what a lot of these
exercises are. I recommend you do a Google or YouTube
search (on exercise names you don't know) before you begin
so you can seamlessly complete the workout. Google Images
is also a great way to see pictures of the exercise. My clients
have enjoyed seeing amazing results and I hope you will too!

O-D STUDIO'S Featured Workouts

The Freshman

This is a basic workout I designed for people who are just starting to work out.

(Repeat 2 - 3 X)

Warm-up - walk 3 minutes at 4.0mph/incline of 4.0

Stretch

10 reverse lunges
10 jumping jacks
10 side lunges

Run 3 minutes at 6.0mph
10 squats
5 push-ups
10 sit-ups
10 dips

Bike 5 minutes at level 5
10 military presses - 5 – 10lbs
10 side lat raises - 5 – 10lbs
Stretch

Walk 3 minutes at 4.0mph/incline of 5.0

The Mommy Clique

I designed this workout for the busy moms. Every city has mommy cliques. They often meet at the park while their kids are playing but end up doing a lot of fitness activities together like yoga or Pilates classes.

(Repeat 3 -5 X)

Warm-up - 3 minutes (bike, treadmill, elliptical or jump rope)
Stretch

15 jumping jacks
5 push-ups
10 v-ups
10 crunches
5 squats one leg up (right and left)
10 leg lifts
10 knee to chest
5 curls with curl bar
5 front press over-hand with curl bar
5 dips

Walk 3 minutes at 4.0mph/incline 7.5
15 squat jumps
Bicycles 30 seconds
10 straddle sit-ups
10 chops with ball or cable

Run 5 minutes at 6.0mph
5 push-ups
Plank 30 seconds
15 hip raises
Flutter kicks 30 seconds

Walk 3 minutes at 4.0mph/incline 7.5
Stretch

The Rabbi

I created this workout for one of my clients who is a Rabbi. This workout is geared for a man over the age of 60. It's not too hard or too easy.

(Repeat 3 X)

Warm-up - 3 minutes

Stretch

10 sit-ups
15 push-ups
10 squats (no weight)
10 military presses (light weight)
10 curls (light weight)
10 pull-ups assisted

Bike 5 minutes
Stretch
10 lunges
15 jumping jacks
10 seated rows

Bike 5 minutes at level 4

The Randi

The Randi was named after a client that is a mom. We soon discovered that she was really born to be a fighter.

(Repeat 3 X)

Warm-up - jump rope 3 minutes

Stretch

15 v-ups
10 push-ups
10 flys - 10lbs
10 round house kicks
10 leg lifts
10 punches (both jabs and strong punches)
15 flutter kicks

Bike 3 minutes
Mountain climbers 30 seconds
15 squat jumps
15 reverse crunches
15 military presses with medicine ball - 10 - 15lbs
10 pull-ups
Jump rope 3 minutes
5 dips
10 punches (both jabs and strong punches)
10 kicks (roundhouse, Muay Thai, sidekicks)
5 push-ups

Run 3 minutes at 6.5mph
15 curls with bar
10 hammer curls
Punches and kicks 3 minutes
Stretch

The Agent

I designed this workout for a client who is a talent agent. The goal is to try this 3 times and live. Personally, this is one of the hardest workouts I have done. It really will make anyone sweat and sore the next few days— if you do not quit half way through.

Warm-up - run 1/2 mile at 6.0mph

Stretch

15 squats with military presses - dumbbell 15lbs
10 pull-ups close grip
10 reverse pull-ups wide grip
10 chin-ups
15 dips
15 decline push-ups
15 incline push-ups
15 barbell dead lifts - 50lbs
15 bent over row - 50lbs

Run 1/2 mile at 6.5mph
15 reverse curls - barbell 25lbs
15 hammer curls - dumbbells 15lb
15 upright rows - barbell 25lbs
15 full boxer sit-ups
15 double crunch

Bike 3 minutes level 5
15 clean and press - barbell 50lb
15 side lateral raises - dumbbells 15lb
15 regular push-ups

Run 1/2 mile at 6.5mph

The Director's Cut

(Repeat 3 X)

Warm-up - bike 5 minutes

Drink a double shot of espresso

Stretch

25 push-ups
10 sit-ups
15 shoulder press - 15lbs dumbbells

Bike 3 mins
5 pull-ups
10 knee to chest
15 arm curls - 15lbs db
5 close grip pull-ups

Jump rope 3 mins
25 decline push-ups
15 shoulder shrugs - 20lbs db
10 squats with front press with barbell - 20lbs
10 side lateral raises - 10lbs db
15 full leg lifts
stretch

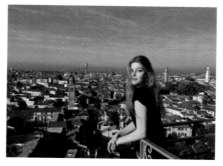

In Milan with Model Zuza K.

The Tom Brady

I designed this workout for my client Tom Brady. It's all about abs and cardio because I did not want to touch his golden arm.

(Repeat 3 - 5 X)

Warm-up - bike 5 minutes

Stretch - especially abs and lower back

15 full leg lifts
15 hip raises
Roll x (bicycles) 30 seconds
15 oblique sit-ups (each side)
Sprint 1 minute at 10.0mph
15 v-ups
20 wood chops with 10lb ball
15 windshield wipers
Sprint 1 minute 10.0mph
Flutter kicks 1 minute
15 stability ball roll outs
Rocks 30 seconds (side to side with resistance band)
15 sit up to a stand
Plank 30 seconds
Sprint 1 minute at 10mph
15 hanging knee to chest
L - hang 30 seconds
15 toe touches (from a hang)
Plank 30 seconds (side plank arm extended both sides - 1 min total)
Sprint 1 minute 10.mph
Stretch
5 min cool down - bike level 3

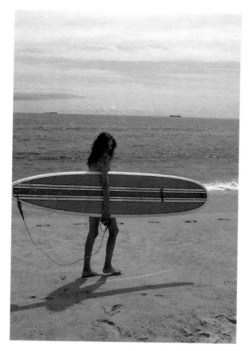

Surf lesson with Model Julia Oberda

Supermodel Workouts

Models are instructed to workout 3 - 6 times per week to get ready for the catwalk. They must eat lean vegetable meals and drink a lot of water mixed with some juice.

The Ultimate Fashion Week Workout

Warm-up - 5 minutes (bike, jump rope, treadmill or elliptical)

Stretch

(Repeat 3 X)

10 push-ups
15 squat jumps
10 leg lifts
10 crunches

Run 3 minutes at 6.0mph
10 side lateral raises - 5 - 10lbs
10 shoulder presses - 5lbs
15 bicep curls
Jump rope 3 minutes
15 donkey kicks (each leg)
5 wide assisted pull-ups
15 sit-ups

Elliptical 3 minutes
15 dancer leaps
15 flutter kicks
Scissors 30 seconds

Bike 3 minutes
15 hip raises
5 push-ups
10 frog jumps
15 sit-ups with hip raise
Stretch
Run/walk 10 minutes (1 minute intervals)

The Runway

This workout is designed to get the girls ready for the runway.

(Repeat 3 X)

Warm-up - 5 minutes – use any cardio machine

Stretch - top to bottom

10 push-ups - 2 sets
15 squat jumps - 2 sets
25 crunches
25 knee to chest or reverse crunches
Treadmill run 3 minutes at 6.5mph
12 side lateral raises - 5lb dumbbells - 2 sets
12 shoulder presses - 5lb dumbbells - 2 sets
12 bicep curls - 5lb dumbbells - 2 sets
Elliptical 3 minutes on level 5
15 dips - 2 sets
5 pull-ups - 2 sets
15 full sit-ups - 2 sets
15 donkey kicks each leg - 2 sets
Scissors 1 minute
15 hip raises - 2 sets
Jump rope 3 minutes
15 frog jumps - 2 sets
15 dancer leaps - 2 sets
15 lunges each leg - 2 sets
15 sumo squats - 2 sets

Run 3 minutes at 7.5mph
Stretch

At the Beach

6 Weeks to a Beach Body

This is a 6 week program you can follow week by week. Try to work out in the morning.

*Once you start, don't take more than a 30 - 45 second rest between sets. The goal is to keep your heart rate up and have it stay in a moderate to high range (doing cardio and weights together will give you that extra push you need to lose weight and strengthen your muscular system).

How it works:

1. Pick 6 exercises each day to do off of *The List*. Don't pick the same exercise twice in a 2 day period. Also one day a week is all cardio (jump rope, bike, run, or swim).

2. Pick any additional daily workout from the following sections:

At the Beach
At Home
At the Park
At the Pool
In your Hotel
In the Office
Strength Training with Weights
At the Gym
Plyometrics
All Cardio Days

68

The List

(Pick 6 each day)

15 - 20 crunches - 2 sets
15 v-ups - 2 sets
Jump rope 3 minutes
12 push-ups - 2 sets
12 dips - 2 sets
Treadmill run 3 minutes at 5mph
15 knee to chest - 2 sets
12 oblique sit-ups each side - 2 sets
Jump rope 3 minutes
12 dumbbell fly's - 10lbs - 2 sets
12 incline presses - 10lbs - 2 sets
15 sit-ups
Quick stretch (lower back especially)
Treadmill run 3 minutes at 5.5mph
15 squats (no weights, arms held out in front of you, head up) - 2 sets
15 lunges each side - 2 sets
30 calf raises
Quick Stretch (hamstrings, quads and calves)
Bike 3 minutes
5 - 8 pull-ups - 2 sets
12 hammer curls - 10lbs - 2 sets
12 dumbbells curls - 10lbs - 2 sets
Jumping jacks 2 minutes
12 seated rows - 20lbs - 2 sets
12 side lateral raises - 5 – 8lbs - 2 sets
12 military presses - 5 - 8lbs - 2 sets
Treadmill run 10 minutes at 6mph
Jump rope 1 minute
Jumping jacks 1 minute
Bike 5 minutes (cool down)
Stretch

The Beach Workout #1:

This is a workout I used to do with my lifeguard crew. Do it at the beach when it's not too crowded. When swimming, you only really need to be in waist-high water. Be safe and don't swim out to sea. Be parallel to the shore, within sight of the lifeguard, and take your time.

Place a flag about 40 yards away from the lifeguard chair.

(Repeat 10 X)

Warm-up - 5 minutes cardio

Stretch

Swim (in waist high water from flag to lifeguard chair)
High knees (run all the way back to the flag you started at)
10 push-ups
10 sit-ups
Beach crawls (lifeguard chair to flag - sprint back to lifeguard chair)
Breast stroke (from flag to lifeguard chair)
Run 10 sprints (from lifeguard chair to flag)

The Beach Workout #2:

(Repeat 3 X)

Warm-up - 5 minutes cardio

Stretch

10 push-ups (face the water for a decline - face away from the water for an incline)
Sand jog - 30 to 40 yards (then jog back)
10 sit-ups (with your back to the water so that you have a decline for added resistance)
Sand lunges - 30 to 40 yards
10 incline push-ups
Sand jog – 30 to 40 yards (then jog back)

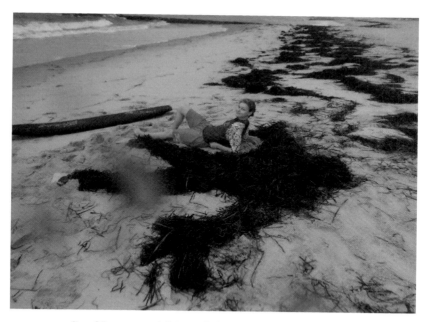

Surf lesson with Model Zuzanna Kaczmarek

The Beach Workout #3

(Repeat 3 X)

Warm-up - 5 minutes jump rope or lite jog

Stretch - 5 - 10 minutes - total body

Legs:

- 15 squats (quads, hamstrings, gluts)
- 15 jumps (in the sand - builds quads and calves)
- 15 vertical jumps/hops (try to get as high as you can)
- 15 sprints in sand
-15 sprints (waist high in the water - rock/rope for more resistance or use bands)
- 15 bear crawl 20 yards
-15 lunges each leg

1 mile run (soft sand)

Abs:

- 25 crunches
- 25 full sit-ups (dig a hole in the sand for both legs to hold your feet - hips stay on the ground)

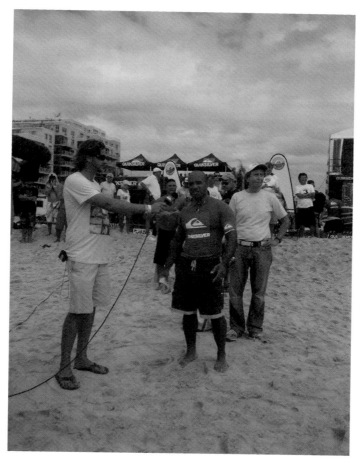

Oscar at Quicksilver Pro Surf Competition

At Home

Equipment you may need for some of the at home workouts include: a pull-up bar, jump rope, exercise ball and free weights.

The O-Diesel 32

This is a 32 minute total body workout. Do each exercise for 1 minute and take no rest between sets.

Warm-up - 5 minutes cardio

Stretch

1. Jumping Jacks
2. Push-ups
3. Sit-ups (arms across your chest)
4. Leg lifts
5. Close grip pull-ups
6. Jump rope
7. Dips
8. Triangle push-ups
9. Squat pops
10. Lunges (alternate legs)
11. Plank
12. Regular push-ups
13. Mountain climbers
14. Shoulder push-ups
15. High knees
16. Pull-ups
17. Decline push-ups
18. Knee to chest
19. Double crunch
20. Sit up to stand
21. Stairs (1 flight)
22. Incline push-ups
23. Chin-ups
24. Scissor kicks
25. Squat thrusts
26. Plank (reach out)
27. Plank (reach up)
28. Roll x crunches
29. Hand stand arch-ups
30. Wall hold
31. Oblique crunch (30 seconds right and left)
32. Behind the neck pull-up

The Lock Up

(Repeat 3 X)

Stretch

15 push-ups

Run in place (high knees) 3 minutes
10 pull-ups
5 close grip chin-ups
15 squats

Run 5 minutes in place high knees
15 sit-ups
15 crunches
15 push-ups

Run 3 minutes in place high knees
15 lunges
10 squat jumps
10 triangle push-ups
10 wide push-ups
10 fingertip push-ups
10 knee-ups

Jumping jacks 3 minutes
15 sit-ups
15 knee to chest
5 close grip chin-ups
10 pull-ups

Jumping jacks 3 minutes
Stretch

Rebound

(Repeat 4 X)

Warm-up - 5 minutes cardio

Stretch

25 clock push-up
25 plyo push-up
25 block push-up
25 wall push-up
25 dive bombs
25 push-up knee to chest
25 push-up side raise
25 push-up one arm leg raise
25 spidermans
25 stagger push-up
25 step-ups
25 Sumo's - after each push up raise on arm up and to the side
(left then right)
Stretch

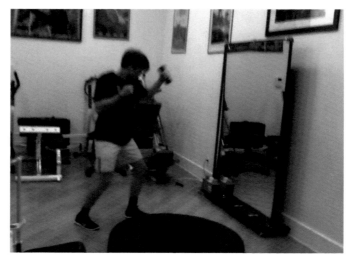

Tech wiz the Cali kid Ryan

30 Seconds

(Repeat 3 - 5 X)

Warm-up - 5 minutes cardio

Stretch

30 Seconds for each:

Jump rope
Up-downs (squat thrust)
Push-ups
Crunches
Squats
Mountain climbers
Pop-ups
Pull-ups
Sit-ups
Jumping jacks
Triangle push-ups
Close grip pull-ups
Burpies
Sprints
Bicycles
Front kicks – alternating legs (foot above the chest)
Decline push-ups
V-ups
Jump rope
Stretch

Legs and Abs at Home

(Repeat 2 X with no rest in between - complete 5 X per week)

Warm-up - 25 jumping jacks

Stretch - hold each for 15 seconds

Wall sit 30 seconds
25 jump squats
20 alternating lunges
40 donkey kicks (20 each leg - hands on the wall - knee to chest then kick straight back)
15 full leg lifts
25 crunches
15 full sit-ups

Stairs 3 minutes (one flight of stairs - knees up high, when coming back down EASY JOG)
50 side lateral leg lifts (25 each side - stand with one hand against the wall, the other on your hips)
25 double crunches
25 jumping jacks
Stretch

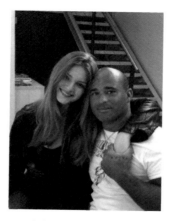

Oscar with model Mayara Rubik

At the Park

The Park Workout

Warm-up - 5 minutes cardio

Stretch

10 dips (on park bench)
10 incline push-ups (on bench)
10 knees to chest (on bench)
10 step-ups (on bench each leg)
10 decline push-ups (feet on bench)
10 bench walks (hands on bench, feet on ground - walk hand to hand length of bench)
10 squat jump pops (on bench)
Flutter kicks 30 seconds (on bench)
5 pull-ups (monkey bars or single bar)
5 chin-ups
10 bench sprints (run as fast as you can to the next bench, then walk back)

Time = 45 minutes to 1 hour

Warm-up - 5 minutes cardio

Stretch

Pull-ups:

20 close grip
20 wide grip
20 behind neck
20 chin-ups
20 hammer grip

Push-ups:

100 regular
100 tricep push ups
100 incline
100 decline

100 dips

100 knees to chest (from a hang)

Goal it to do the total workout in 32 minutes

The Runner

Warm-up - 5 minutes cardio

Stretch

1 mile run
10 push-ups
10 - 15 yard sprints
10 push-ups
Stretch
10 - 15 yard sprints
10 push-ups
10 sit-ups

Mile run
5 push-ups
Mountain climbers 1 minute
5 squat pops
Mountain climbers 30 seconds
10 sit-ups

10 - 50 yard sprints (5 push-ups and 5 sit-ups after each sprint)
2 mile run (easy pace)
Stretch

Burn baby burn

Warm-up - 5 minutes cardio

Stretch - hamstrings, calves, lower back

10 bullet lunges
10 around the worlds
10 pop-ups
10 reverse lunges
10 jumping jacks
10 scales (front and back)
10 leaps
10 hurdles
10 side lunges
10 steps-ups with a twist
10 frog jumps
10 front kicks
10 sprints
10 squats
10 squats with calf lifts
10 flutter kicks on floor
10 side leg raises (both legs on floor)
10 big circles on floor
10 rebounds
Run 5 minutes
Stretch

The Poopa

Warm-up - 5 minutes cardio

Stretch

15 lunges each leg
15 squats - 10lbs
15 pop-ups squat to a jump
15 leg curls - 15lbs
15 leg extensions -15lbs
20 reverse lunges - alt legs
Mountain climbers 30 seconds
Stairs 1 minute or one flight
10 wind sprints
Bike 3 minutes
Squat thrusts 30 seconds

Jump ½ half turns right to left then left to right - 1 minute
Super girl 1 minute (up and down)
Side step 1 minute (right then left)

Run in place 1 minute (as fast as you can)
15 side lat leg kicks - each side
15 diving kicks - like you are kicking a field goal or soccer ball
Tuck jumps 1 minute

15 reverse supergirls (tummy on the stability ball at your waist
with legs straight and hands in front. Drive your heels up to
the ceiling and toes back to touch the floor)
Stretch

The Running Back

(Repeat 3 - 5 X)

Warm-up - 1 mile run

Stretch

Jumping jacks 30 seconds
Push-up pops 30 seconds
10 yard sprints with high knees 30 seconds
Side to side lateral drills 30 seconds
15 single leg jumps (each leg)

Half jump turns 30 seconds - shoulder apart and jump right
then left then left then right
Blocks 30 seconds
Double jumps 1 minute
Stairs 3 minutes up and down
Around the world push-ups 1 minute
Hops 30 seconds
15 box jumps
Scales to a jump front and back single leg jumps
15 dead lifts - 50 to 100lbs

Throws against wall 1 minute - with a 25lb ball squat then on
the way up toss the ball to the ceiling and make sure you catch
it
Single leg hops with rings or latter 1 minute
1 mile run

The Outdoors #1

Warm-up - 5 minutes cardio

Stretch

Jump rope 3 minutes
15 sit-ups
15 crunches
15 v-ups
15 roll x bicycles
15 oblique's - one hand behind your head and the other on the floor or grass the elbow to the knee then repeat to the other side switch arms
15 leg lifts

Jump rope 3 minutes
10 push-ups
10 incline push-ups
10 decline push-ups
10 rocks
10 dips
10 pop-ups

Jump rope 5 minutes
15 squats
15 lunges
15 pop-ups
15 mountain climbers
15 jumping jacks
10 squat thrusts

Jump rope 5 minutes
10 sprints
15 mountain climbers
15 front kicks (each leg)

Jump rope 3 minutes
Stretch

Warm-up - 5 minutes cardio

Stretch

Run 5 minutes
Push-ups 3 minutes
Jump rope 3 minutes
Bike 5 minutes

Sit-ups 3 minutes
Jumping jacks 3 minutes
Wide grip pull-ups 3 minutes
Bike 5 minutes

Squats/pop-ups/lunges 3 minutes - sets of 10
Run 3 minutes
Sit-ups/crunches/leg lifts/roll x 2 minutes - sets of 10
Jump rope 1 minute
Bike 3 minutes

Chin-ups 1 minute
Tri push-ups 1 minute
Sprints 10 yards 1 minute
Stretch

At the Pool

Pool Workout #1

(Repeat 10X)

Swim 1 lap freestyle (run back)
Swim 2 laps breaststroke
Swim 2 laps freestyle (run 2 laps)
Swim 1 lap backstroke (run 4 laps)
Swim 2 laps breaststroke
Swim 2 laps freestyle

Run 6 laps as fast as you can
Swim 2 laps as fast as you can

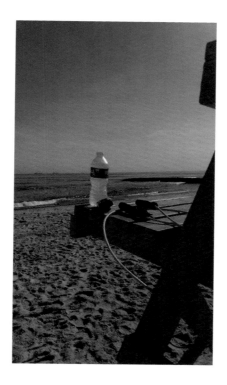

Pool Workout #2

(Try to Repeat 2 X)

- 25 dips
- 25 push-ups
- 25 decline push-ups (feet up on a sand mound)
- 25 diamond triangle push-ups
- 25 close grip push-ups - hand under shoulders

Swim laps for 30 minutes (your arms are going to feel like a boat anchor) then do it all again.

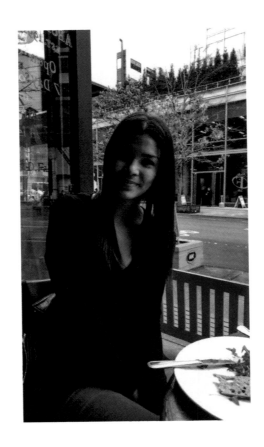

Lunch in SoHo with Model Louisa Taadou

In your Hotel

Hotel Workout

Stretch
Jumping jacks 1 minute
10 dips
10 sit-ups
10 push-ups
Rebounds on bed 30 seconds (sit on the bed then get up as fast as you can)
10 lunges
10 squats
10 chair push-ups hands on the back of the chair

Jump rope
10 v-ups
10 decline push-ups feet on the chair hands on the floor
10 triangle push-up
Stand to plank walk your hands down to a push up position from a standing position
15 pop-ups lying on the floor try to get up as fast as you can
Jumping jacks 1 minute
10 crunches
10 leg lifts
10 oblique crunches - each side
Stretch

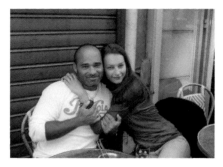
Oscar with model Vanessa Perron in Paris

In the Office

The Office Workout

In your chair:

Abs (Repeat 3 X)
Contract your stomach and hold for 10, 15, 20 seconds etc.
The longer you hold the stronger your stomach will become.

Knees to chest - 2 sets of 10 reps
In your office chair, using your arms to help support you, hold
the side of the chair and extend your legs out – then bring them
back to into your chest if possible.

Using your chair or end of your desk:

Arm dips - 2 sets of 10 reps
Extend your legs out so that you are doing a release lean on the
desk or chair.

Arm curls - 2 sets of 10 reps
Using a book /water bottle - firm grip on the open ends - curls
(bring arms up - both at same time squeeze the muscle
(contract)

Chest - push-ups - 2 sets of 10 reps

Legs - squats 10 reps

Shoulders - side lateral raises, and military presses using a book or a water bottle - 15 reps

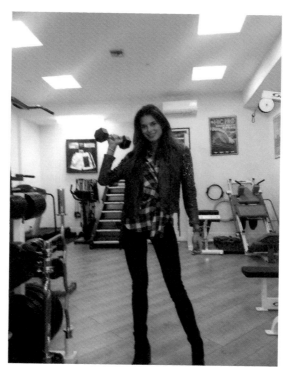

Model Raica Oliveira at O-D Studio

At the Gym

O-Diesel Abs

Warm-up - 5 minutes cardio

Stretch

15 leg lifts
15 combo crunch with knee to chest
30 roll x (bicycles)
Plank 30 seconds
15 oblique sit-ups
15 v-ups
15 hanging knee to chest
Side plank 30 seconds (each side)
Sit-up rocks (each side)
Side to side 30 seconds
15 standing oblique side to side - 10 - 15lbs
15 chops with exercise ball - 10lbs
15 hip raises
20 scissor kicks
15 stability ball - feet on the ball hand on the floor - roll the
ball out from your chest till your legs are straight then back to
your knees to your chest
15 weight crunches 10lbs, 25lbs
Flutter kicks 30 seconds
15 dumbbell crunch on arm - 10lb
30 hanging side to side - knee to chest
Lying windshield wiper on your back legs in the air hands at
your side - let your legs swing side to side try touching the
floor but keep them together
15 oblique crunches - each side

Bootcamp

(Repeat 3 X)

Warm-up - 5 minutes cardio

Stretch

Run 3 minutes 6.0 mph
10 push-ups
10 jumping jacks
15 squats
10 push-ups
10 dips
10 jumping jacks
10 squat jumps
10 military presses
10 push-ups
15 sit-ups
15 leg lifts
10 squat thrusts

Run 3 minutes at 6.0mph
10 pull-ups wide grip
3 - 8 close grip pull-ups
10 side lat raises - 5 - 25lbs
10 curls - 25 - 50lbs
10 jumping jacks
Mountain climbers 30 seconds
10 push-ups
15 sit-ups
Jump rope 3 minutes
15 leg lifts
15 knee to chest
15 bicycle crunches
Stretch

Legs and Abs – Gym Workout

(Repeat 2 X with no rest in between - complete 5 X per week)

Warm-up - 5 minutes cardio

Stretch

10 minute walk at 4.0mph/incline of 5.0
10 girl push-ups on knees
15 lunges
10 squat jumps

Run 3 minutes at 6.0mph
10 full sit-ups
15 crunches
10 leg lifts
25 jumping jacks

Run 3 minutes at 6.5mph
10 girl push-ups
10 hip raises
25 jumping jacks

Run 3 minutes at 6.5mph
10 dips
10 sit-ups
10 squat jumps

Walk 5 minutes at 4.0mph/incline 8.0
Stretch

Gym blast back and arms

Warm-up - 5 minutes jump rope

Stretch

Back: **(Repeat X 2)**
- 10 pull-ups wide grip
- 10 rows - 50lbs
- 10 lat pull-downs in front
- 10 lat pull-downs back
- 10 close grip pull-downs

Run 2 miles at 6.5mph

Arms: **(Repeat X 2)**
- 15 barbell curls - 20lbs
- 15 hammer curls – 15-25lbs dumbbell
- 15 concentration curls – 25-50lbs curl bar
- 15 tri push-downs - 40 - 60lbs
- 15 reverse curls - 40 - 60lbs
- 5 close grip pull-ups

Bike 5 minutes at level 6
Jump rope 3 minutes
Stretch

Gym Blast Abs and Shoulders

Warm-up - 5 minutes jump rope

Stretch

Shoulders: **(Repeat X 2)**
- 12 side lateral raises - 15lbs
- 12 military presses with bar - 20lbs
- 12 shrugs - 30lbs dumbbell
- 12 upright rows - 15lbs dumbbell
- 12 front lateral raises - 25lb plate
- 12 front press - 25lb plate

Bike 3 minutes level 7
Run 5 minutes at 6.5mph
Jump rope 1 minute

Core and Legs: **(Repeat X 2)**
- 15 knee to chest
- 15 leg lifts
- 15 sit up to stand
- 15 squat thrusts

Bicycle 30 seconds
Plank 30 seconds

Run 3 minutes at 7.0mph at incline level 5

Chest

Warm-up - 5 minutes cardio

Stretch

10 flat bench (light, medium, light, heavy) - 4 sets
10 incline bench (light, medium, light, heavy) - 4 sets
10 fly decline bench (light, medium, light, heavy) - 4 sets
10 decline bench – 4 sets
30 reverse dips -4 sets
10 pull-overs (light, medium, light, heavy) - 4 sets
10 close grip press- bar only - 5 sets
15 tri-push-ups
Stretch

Shoulders

Warm-up - 5 minutes cardio

Stretch

10 shrugs (light, medium, light, heavy) - 4 sets
10 military presses (light, medium, light, heavy) - 4 sets
10 side lat raises (light, medium, light, heavy) - 4 sets
10 front lat raises (light, medium, light, heavy) - 4 sets
10 upright rows (light, medium, light, heavy) - 4 sets
10 military presses behind the neck (light, medium, light, heavy) - 4 sets
10 squat presses (light, medium, light, heavy) - 4 sets
15 deltoid dips (light, medium, light, heavy) - 3 sets

Kick Box

(Repeat the following between 2 – 5 X)

Warm-up - 3 minute jump rope

Stretch

10 front kicks each leg
10 up-downs
10 roundhouse kicks
10 squats
10 Muay Thai kicks
10 jabs alternating sides
10 sit-ups
10 hooks alternating sides
10 alternating punches (right and left)
10 v-ups
Punching and kicking on bag 3 minutes
10 upper cuts with jabs
Just kicks 3 minutes
Just punches 3 minutes
Jump rope 3 minutes

10 elbows (right and left)
10 sidekicks (right and left)
10 knees (right and left)

3 minutes of combos:

Combo 1: 1, 2, front kick, elbow
Combo 2: jab, knee, elbow, hook to body
Combo 3: 1, 2 hook, roundhouse, uppercut
Combo 4: roundhouse, Muay Thai kick, cross, hook
Combo 5: cross (right), cross (left), sidekick jab, jab then uppercut

Rope and Arms

Warm-up - 5 minutes (bike, treadmill or jump rope)

Stretch

Do between each arm exercise:

1. **1 X climb rope**
2. **5 push-ups**

10 curls with weight
10 hammer curls with weight
10 tri push-downs with weight
10 tri extensions with weight
10 reverse curls with weight
10 dips (no weight)
10 wide grip curls with weight
10 alt dumbbell curls w/ twist with weight

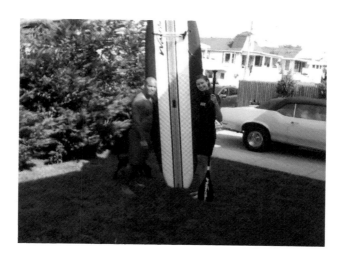

Standup paddle lesson with Oscar and model Kasia Krol

Quick Power

Warm up - 5 minutes cardio

Stretch

10 pull-ups with leg raise
10 squat military presses
15 pull-ups close grip
15 pull-ups wide grip
15 pull-ups reverse grip
15 dips
15 decline push-ups
15 push-up to a single leg raise
15 dumbbell curl to overhand press
15 barbell dead lift
15 bent over row (barbell)

Run 1 mile

15 barbell upright row - 25lbs
10 front lat raise barbell only

Bike 3 miles or run ½ mile run

15 clean and jerk to a press barbell - 50lbs
15 reverse curls curl bar - 20lbs
10 wide grip pull-ups
10 wide grip chin-ups

Abs, that's all

Stretch, especially lower back

15 crunches (legs up in the air)
15 hip raises (lying on back, feet apart)
30 second rock and roll with ball 1 minute
15 v-ups
15 single leg lifts with a hip raise
15 sit-ups
15 leg lifts (both)

Bicycles 1 minute
15 knees to chest

Flutter kicks 1 minute
15 reverse crunch
15 straddle sit-ups with twist
15 dumbbell reach
15 pike dumbbell reach

Rope climb
15 wood Chops with ball or cable
15 reverse chop
Side plank 1 minute each side
Walk 5 minute at 4.0speed highest incline

+Body Blast

Warm up - 5 minutes cardio

Stretch

100 incline push-ups
10 jump to pull-up - 3 sets
15 dips - 3 sets
10 knee to chest - 3 sets
15 incline fly's - 10 - 25lbs

Run stairs 3 minutes
10 full leg lifts (from a hanging position)

Walk 3 minutes at 4.0mph incline at 5
5 close grip pull-ups - 3sets
5 wide grip pull-ups with assistance - 3 sets
Last set decline push-ups to 100
15 reps Rows 3sets 15 -50lbs

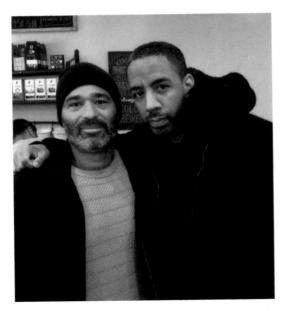

Oscar and R&B singer and Producer Ryan Leslie

Cardio + Upper Body

Warm up - 5 minutes cardio

Stretch

Run 1 mile at 6.0 - 7.0mph
15 dips - 4 sets
Bench press 15 to 25 reps bar only
Bike 1 minute at level 10
10 close grip pull-ups - 3 sets

Walk 3 minutes/incline of 15 at 4.0 speed
10 jump pull-ups - 3 sets

Run 1 set of stairs 3 minutes

Bike 1 minute at level 13
15 sit-ups 3 sets

Bike 1 minute at level 13
15 curls 25lbs barbell or dumbbells 3sets

Bike 1 minute at level 8
15 crunches 3 sets
25 push-ups 3sets
25 decline push up 3 sets
25 front shoulder presses with the bar 3sets
Stretch

Back and chest, Cardio Workout

Warm-up - 5 minutes cardio

Stretch

25 push-ups

Run ½ mile at 6.0mph
10 lat pull-downs F/B/Chin - 75lbs

Run ½ mile at 6.5mph
10 - 15 lat pull-downs F/B/Chin - 75lbs
25 push-ups
Plank 1 minute

Run ½ mile at 7.0mph
25 push-ups
Jump rope 3 minutes

10 close grip lat pull-down F/B/Chin - 100lbs
10 decline push-ups
15 seated rows - 75lbs
25 decline push-ups
15 seated rows - 75lbs
Run 3 minutes at 6.0mph
Stretch

Shadow Box Cardio

(Repeat 5 X)

Warm up - 5 minutes jump rope

Stretch

Shadow box 3 minutes
Jump rope 3 minutes
15 round house kicks to bag or pads - left than right side
Jump rope 3 minutes
Shadow box 3 minutes
Jump rope 3 minutes
Punches and kicks to bag or pads 5 minutes
Stretch work on your splits

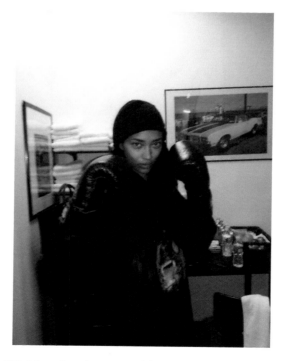

Kickboxing lesson with model Anais Mali

Strength Training with Weights

Chest with Weights

Warm up - 5 minutes cardio

Stretch

5 sets bench (15 light, 15 light, 3 – 8 heavy, 10 light, 3 – 5 heavy)
5 sets incline (15 light, 15 light, 3 – 8 heavy, 10 light, 3 – 5 heavy)
5 sets decline (15 light, 15 light, 3 – 8 heavy, 10 light, 3 – 5 heavy)
5 sets fly (15 light, 15 light, 3 – 8 heavy, 10 light, 3 – 5 heavy)
5 sets dips (with weight) (15 light, 15 light, 3 – 8 heavy, 10 light, 3 – 5 heavy)

Pull-overs
5 sets DB press incline (15 light, 15 light, 3 – 8 heavy, 10 light, 3 – 5 heavy)
5 sets pec deck (fly) (15 light, 15 light, 3 – 8 heavy, 10 light, 3 – 5 heavy)
Stretch

Shoulders with Weights

Warm up - 5 min cardio

Stretch

5 sets military press behind the neck (15 light, 15 light, 5 – 8 heavy, 10 light, 3 – 5 heavy)
5 sets upright rows (15 light, 15 light, 5 – 8 heavy, 10 light, 3 – 5 heavy)
5 sets shrugs (15 light, 15 light, 5 – 8 heavy, 10 light, 3 – 5 heavy)
5 sets side lateral raises (15 light, 15 light, 5 – 8 heavy, 10 light, 3 – 5 heavy)
5 sets military press front (15 light, 15 light, 5 – 8 heavy, 10 light, 3 – 5 heavy)
5 sets hammer curl to front press (15 light, 15 light, 5 – 8 heavy, 10 light, 3 – 5 heavy)
5 sets DB peck press (15 light, 15 light, 5 – 8 heavy, 10 light, 3 – 5 heavy)
5 sets bent over side lateral raise (15 light, 15 light, 5 – 8 heavy, 10 light, 3 – 5 heavy)
5 sets front overhead raise (15 light, 15 light, 5 – 8 heavy, 10 light, 3 – 5 heavy)
Stretch

Arms with Weights

Warm up - 5 min cardio

Stretch

5 sets hammer curls (15 light, 15 light, 5 – 8 heavy, 10 light, 3 – 5 heavy)
5 sets curls (15 light, 15 light, 5 – 8 heavy, 10 light, 3 – 5 heavy)
5 sets wide grip curls (15 light, 15 light, 5 – 8 heavy, 10 light, 3 – 5 heavy)
5 sets DB alt curls (15 light, 15 light, 5 – 8 heavy, 10 light, 3 – 5 heavy)
5 sets tri extensions (15 light, 15 light, 5 – 8 heavy, 10 light, 3 – 5 heavy)
5 sets tri push downs (15 light, 15 light, 5 – 8 heavy, 10 light, 3 – 5 heavy)5 sets reverse curls (15 light, 15 light, 5 – 8 heavy, 10 light, 3 – 5 heavy)
5 sets reverse curls with rope (15 light, 15 light, 5 – 8 heavy, 10 light, 3 – 5 heavy)
5 sets preacher curls (15 light, 15 light, 5 – 8 heavy, 10 light, 3 – 5 heavy)
10 pull-ups with added weight
5 sets tri extensions with rope (15 light, 15 light, 5 – 8 heavy, 10 light, 3 – 5 heavy)
Stretch

Back with Weights

Warm up - 5 min cardio

Stretch

5 sets lat pulldowns front (15 light, 15 light, 5 – 8 heavy, 10 light, 3 – 5 heavy)

5 sets lat pulldowns back (15 light, 15 light, 5 – 8 heavy, 10 light, 3 – 5 heavy)

5 sets row (15 light, 15 light, 5 – 8 heavy, 10 light, 3 – 5 heavy)5 sets bent over rows (15 light, 15 light, 5 – 8 heavy, 10 light, 3 – 5 heavy)

5 sets bent over rows reverse grip (15 light, 15 light, 5 – 8 heavy, 10 light, 3 – 5 heavy)

5 sets one arm rows (15 light, 15 light, 5 – 8 heavy, 10 light, 3 – 5 heavy)

5 sets close grip pull downs (15 light, 15 light, 5 – 8 heavy, 10 light, 3 – 5 heavy)

5 sets dead lifts (15 light, 15 light, 5 – 8 heavy, 10 light, 3 – 5 heavy)

10 wide grip pull-ups
10 chin-ups
Stretch

Legs with Weight

Warm up - 5 min cardio

Stretch

5 sets squats (15 light, 15 light, 5 – 8 heavy, 10 light, 3 – 5 heavy)

5 sets leg presses (15 light, 15 light, 5 – 8 heavy, 10 light, 3 – 5 heavy)

5 sets leg extensions (15 light, 15 light, 5 – 8 heavy, 10 light, 3 – 5 heavy)

5 sets leg curls (15 light, 15 light, 5 – 8 heavy, 10 light, 3 – 5 heavy)

5 sets calf raises (15 light, 15 light, 5 – 8 heavy, 10 light, 3 – 5 heavy)

5 sets lunges (15 light, 15 light, 5 – 8 heavy, 10 light, 3 – 5 heavy)

5 sets dead lifts alt grip (15 light, 15 light, 5 – 8 heavy, 10 light, 3 – 5 heavy)

5 sets squats (15 light, 15 light, 5 – 8 heavy, 10 light, 3 – 5 heavy)

5 sets farmer walks 10 yards (15 light, 15 light, 5 – 8 heavy, 10 light, 3 – 5 heavy)

Stretch

Plyometrics

Plyometrics

Warm-up - 5 minutes cardio

Stretch especially calves and lower back

Jump rope 3 minute
15 frog jumps
– 2 minutes side to side (shuffle step)
15 jumping jacks
5 - bunny hops 25 yards
15 jump straddle
Step-ups 2 minutes
15 scales front and back
15 single leg broad jumps (right and left)
10 up downs

Burst:
30 sit-ups
30 leg lifts
30 hip-ups
30 oblique's
Mountain climbers 1min
Hurdles jump over 10 yards 3mins
10 step and throw med ball 25lbs (each lega0

Jump rope 2 minutes
5 – Broad jumps
5 – Grapevine 25 yards
15 tuck jumps
15 jump switch ½ turn (both sides)
15 jump-ups (box jumps)
10 sprints 25 yards
Stretch

Legs with Plyo

Warm-up - 5 minutes

Stretch

Jump rope 3 minutes
15 lunges each side - dumbbell 15lb
15 squats - dumbbell 15 - 25lb
Jumps half turn right 30 seconds
Jumps half turn left 30 seconds
Mountain climbers 30 seconds
Squat jumps 30 seconds
15 leg press weight
15 leg extension weight
Jump rope 3 minutes

Shuffle run side to side 30 seconds
15 front kicks each side
Quick feet 30 seconds
15 heavy squats
Jumps full turn right 30 seconds
Jumps full turn left 30 seconds
5 minutes bike level 7
Stretch

All Cardio Days

All Cardio Days:

Warm up - 5 minutes jump rope

Stretch

* **Swim 40 minutes**

* **Bike outdoors 10 miles**

* **Run outdoors 3 to 10 miles**

* **Tennis - 3 sets with 1 mile run after**

* **Jump rope - 45 minutes**

* **Basketball - 5 games of 21**

Triathlon

Warm up - 5 minutes jump rope

Stretch

Swim 30 minutes

Run 3 miles

Bike 10 miles

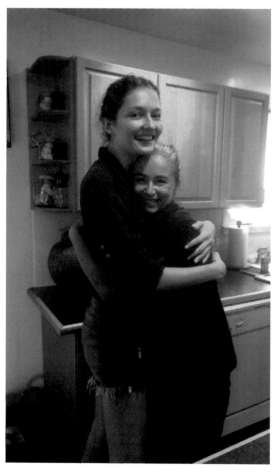

Agnineszka owner of KOYA MGMT with Solange Wilvert

at The Beach House

Extra Workouts

(Repeat X 5)

Warm up - 5 minutes

Stretch

10 push-ups
5 close grip pull-ups
10 dips
15 crunches
15 knees to chest
15 squats
25 sit-ups
25 boxer sit-ups
10 squat jumps
15 jumping jacks
Mountain climbers 15 seconds
5 push-ups
5 wide pull-ups
15 military presses w/ medicine ball
15 leg lifts
Roll x 15 seconds
15 jumping jacks
15 alternative leg lunges
15 squats
10 push-ups
15 knee to chest
8 wide pull-ups
15 crunches
15 leg lifts
15 dips

O-D on the Go

(2 days on, rest, 2 days on)

#1

Warm up - 5 minutes cardio

Stretch

Jump rope 3 minutes
15 push-ups
15 dips
30 jumping jacks
25 crunches
Jump rope 3 minutes
15 squats
15 lunges each leg
15 leg lifts
15 push-ups
15 dips
Jump rope 3 minutes
15 sit-ups
10 reverse crunches
15 dips
15 close grip push-ups
30 jumping jacks
15 lunges
15 leg lifts
Jump rope 3 minutes
Stretch

Warm up - 5 minutes cardio

Stretch

50 jumping jacks
10 leg lifts
10 squats
10 lunges
10 reverse lunges
10 squat thrusts
Mountain climbers 30 seconds
10 frog leaps
50 jumping jacks
Stretch legs/hamstrings/gluts/hips

Complete 3 sets of the following:

10 sit-ups
10 crunches
10 leg lifts
10 planks
10 knees to chest
10 hip raises
10 flutter kicks
10 bicycles
10 crunches
10 rocks

Jump rope 5 minutes
20 seconds high knees
15 squat jumps
15 sit-ups
15 side leg raises (each leg)
Jump rope 3 minutes

Warm up - 5 minutes

Stretch

Jump rope 3 minutes
15 push-ups
15 close grip push-ups
15 wide grip push-ups

Jump rope 3 minutes
10 dips
15 rocks
15 decline push-ups

Jump rope 3 minutes
10 push-up pops
10 push-up to dip cross over rock
15 incline push-ups

Jump rope 3 minutes
10 push-ups on ball single hand
10 hand stands hold each of 3 seconds then down then back up again
10 hand stand push-ups
15 push-up reach

Jump rope 3 minutes

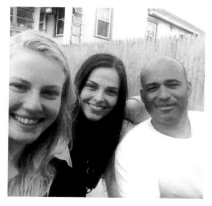

Oscar with models Maxine Schiff and Lisette Van Den Brand

WHAT TO EAT

Below is a list of ideas you can use for various meal times.

Breakfast:

* Cereal (whole grain) w/ soy or real milk

* Egg whites

* Yogurt w/ fruit

* Oatmeal

* Mixed fruit

* Turkey Bacon

* Whole wheat toast

* Veggie omelet

Lunch:

* Fish w/ veggies

* Chicken w/ brown rice

* Lean cut steak w/ veggies

* Mixed green salad/soup

* Wraps – turkey, veggie, tuna – all with veggies and sauce

* ½ cup black beans w/ yellow rice

Dinner:

* Fish w/ brown rice

* Rice and beans

* Whole wheat pasta

* Wrap w/ salad

* Chicken w/ salad

* Meat w/ veggies

Snacks:

* Mixed nuts, fruit, whole wheat crackers, trail mix, raisins, dried fruit, rice crackers, and peanut butter.

** No power or protein bars or shakes.

Drinks:

* Drink as much water, tea and juice as you want – limit coffee, wine (only 1 glass per day).

** No beer or hard drinks.

** Only 1 cup coffee per day.

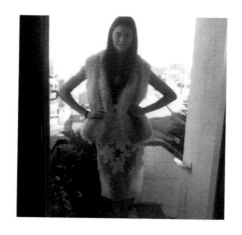

Model Lina Sandberg

TWO WEEK DIET PLAN

Below is an example of how I would recommend someone eat for 2 weeks if they are trying to add a diet change to their workout plan.

Day One:

Breakfast – 1 egg w/ side of mixed greens and water

Snack – ½ cup of mixed nuts with juice

Lunch – Tuna on whole wheat bread with water

Snack – 1 apple with water

Dinner – Brown rice w/ string beans and chicken

Day Two:

Breakfast – Bowl of Cheerios with Fruit

Snack – Yogurt plain

Lunch – Mixed green salad w/ lemon pepper dressing with water

Snack – Banana with water

Dinner – Grilled fish w/ veggies and water

Day Three:

Breakfast – Toast with coffee

Snack – Dried fruit with ½ cup of water

Lunch – Grilled chicken with brown rice

Snack – Apple with water

Dinner – Grilled pork chop w/ side salad and 1 glass of red wine

Day Four:

Breakfast – 2 eggs scrambled w/ scallions and peppers - 1 cup of coffee

Snack – Mixed nuts with ½ cup of juice

Lunch – Grilled chicken salad

Snack – 2 mandarins with water

Dinner – Soup

Day Five:

Breakfast – Yogurt with blueberries and juice

Snack – Trail mix with ½ cup water

Lunch – 1 cup pasta with red sauce

Snack – ½ grapefruit with water

Dinner – Sushi (5 pieces) w/ bowl of brown rice

Day Six:

Breakfast – 1 waffle w/ fruit and juice

Snack – 10 Wheat Thins with juice

Lunch – Chicken fried rice with water

Snack – ½ cup pistachios with juice

Dinner – Salmon w/ steamed veggies and 1 glass of red wine

Day Seven:

Breakfast – 1 egg white with green tea

Snack – 3 full carrots with water

Lunch – Soup

Snack – Pear with water

Dinner – 1 baked potato w/ side salad

Day Eight:

Breakfast – Mix fruit with tea

Snack – Broccoli w/dressing

Lunch – Mix salad with chicken

Snack – ½ cup grapes with water

Dinner – Mixed greens steamed with brown rice

Day Nine:

Breakfast – Oatmeal with cinnamon

Snack – Banana with juice

Lunch – Spinach salad with onions

Snack – Cut carrots w/ oil and vinegar dressing

Dinner – Grilled salmon with steamed broccoli

Day Ten:

Breakfast – 2 eggs over easy with 1 cup coffee

Snack – ½ cup raisins with water

Lunch – Miso soup with tea

Snack – 5 wheat crackers with juice

Dinner – Grilled steak w/ ½ cup rice and 1 glass red wine

Day Eleven:

Breakfast – 1 bowl of cereal – corn flakes with banana

Snack – 5 crackers w/ cheese and juice

Lunch – Chicken w/ rice, peas, and corn

Snack – Apple with water

Dinner – Grilled Shrimp w/ side salad and 1 glass white wine

Day Twelve:

Breakfast – Mixed green salad w/ dressing and juice

Snack – ½ cup of mixed nuts

Lunch – Chicken wrap with water

Snack – Yogurt w/ fruit and juice

Dinner – Mixed greens steamed with brown rice

Day Thirteen:

Breakfast – Wheat toast w/ jam and coffee

Snack – 3 cookies with juice

Lunch – Tuna salad wrap with water

Snack – ½ cup dry Cheerios w/ berries and water

Dinner – Grilled fish w/ veggies and white wine

Day Fourteen:

Breakfast – ½ grapefruit with tea

Snack – Broccoli w/ cauliflower and ½ cup dressing

Lunch – Cheese burger wrap with green tea

Snack – ½ cup mixed nuts with water

Dinner – Grilled chicken w/ ½ cup grilled potatoes

Cheat Day (once a month)

Breakfast – Veggie omelet with juice or coffee

Snack – Coffee with slice of pie

Lunch – Grilled cheese with tea

Snack – 3 cookies with tea

Dinner – Pork chop with brown rice

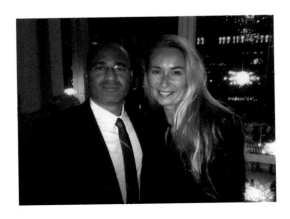

Oscar and his wife AgA

FINAL NOTE FROM OSCAR

If you learn how to cultivate natural strength in your life my promise to you is that your sense of play, enjoyment and life force will return to you. Practice seizing opportunities and learn that it feels good to take care of your body. You will feel good about your ability to focus on your goals and to take risks.

I hope this book has been a guide for you on your journey of fitness. Feel free to contact me with any questions or comments and follow me on social media.

www.O-Dstudio.com

Facebook: O-D studio

Twitter: @O_Diesel

Instagram: Oscar_odstudio